M000159093

The Beginner's Guide to Histamine Intolerance

DR. JANICE JONEJA, PhD

Introduction   v

How to Use This Book   vii

CHAPTER 1: What is Histamine and Histamine Intolerance?   1

Symptoms of Histamine Excess   1
Why Does Too Much Histamine Cause a Problem?   3
How Does the Body Usually get Rid of Histamine?   3
Where is Histamine Found in the Body?   4
Why do Histamine Levels Increase?   4
     Inflammation and allergy   4
     Mastocytosis and MCAD (mast cell activation disorder)   5
     Hormone changes   6
     Medical agents and medicines   6
     Diet   7
How Much Histamine is Too Much?   7
How is Histamine Intolerance Diagnosed?   7
How can you distinguish between Histamine Intolerance and Food Allergy?   8
Where Does Histamine Come from in Food?   9
     Histamine in the ripening of fruits   10
     Histamine caused by incorrect processing of fish or shellfish   10
     Histamine in manufactured foods   11
     Histamine release by natural and artificial chemicals   11
     Histamine derived from foods by unknown mechanisms   12

CHAPTER 2: Managing Histamine Intolerance   13

Is There a Cure for This Illness or is it for Life?   14
How can Diet Help in Reducing Excess Histamine?   15
The Role of Supplements, Probiotics and Antihistamines in Treating Histamine Intolerance   16
     Diamine Oxidase (DAO)   16
     Antihistamines   18
     Stomach Acid Inhibitors   19
     Other supplements   19
The Histamine-Restricted Diet: Foods to Eat, Foods to Avoid   22
     How to follow the diet   22
     General rules, hints and tips for the histamine-restricted diet   23

Safe to eat, foods to avoid: what to eat on the histamine-restricted diet 24

Questions related to the histamine-restricted diet, and other diet programs 36

CHAPTER 3: Other Conditions and Related Information 43

Mastocytosis/Mast Cell Activation Disorder (MCADs) 43

Diabetes 44

Digestive Tract Issues, Diarrhea and IBS 45

CHAPTER 4: Case Studies 47

Anaphylaxis 47

Angioedema ("Swelling Under the Skin") and Urticaria ("Hives") After Food Poisoning 49

Anxiety 52

Dust Mite Allergy and Grief 55

Facial Rash, Low Energy, Burning Eyes, Anxiety Attacks, Hair Loss, Weight Loss and Poor Sleep 57

Fatigue 60

Hormone Fluctuations, Periods and Ovulation ("Time of the Month") 62

Idiopathic Anaphylaxis ("Unknown Allergy") 63

Interstitial Cystitis and Mast Cells 65

Pregnancy 69

Puberty, Headaches and Urticaria ("Hives") 70

Sexual issues: semen allergy and vaginal irritation 72

Urticaria ("Hives"), Stress and Depression 76

About Dr. Janice Vickerstaff Joneja, Ph.D. 81

Further Resources 83

References 85

INDEX 89

INTRODUCTION

I have worked with food allergy for many years and have always been particularly interested in histamine sensitivity.

Although many of my colleagues in both the allergy and the more general medical world continue to deny its existence, as far as I am concerned, histamine sensitivity has always been a very real condition and, since the 1990s, it has been a focus of my research work.

This book will give you a quick overview of the condition and its symptoms which should allow you to work out whether it is the cause your problems. It will then give you details of my histamine-restricted diet—the bedrock of my histamine management program—some interesting case histories and some suggestions for further reading.

If you would like to investigate the condition in detail, and learn about the science, please refer to my book, **"Histamine Intolerance: the Complete Guide for Medical Professionals"**.

But, if you just feel that your symptoms may be caused by histamine intolerance and would like to know what you could do to alleviate them—then read on.

I hope that you find this book helpful.

Janice Vickerstaff Joneja, PhD

February 2017

HOW TO USE THIS BOOK

If you think that your symptoms could be caused by histamine intolerance—or if you believe they are and want to know what to do about it—this book is for you.

However, it is important to remember that the advice given in this book is not a substitute for a consultation with your own doctor or physician; you must first be sure that you do not have an underlying medical problem before you assume that you are histamine intolerant.

If you are seeking help for a child, you must first refer to their medical professional before changing their diet or giving them supplements. It is essential that you get a definitive diagnosis before making assumptions, or starting any kind of treatment, when you are dealing with a child's health.

CHAPTER 1: WHAT IS HISTAMINE AND HISTAMINE INTOLERANCE?

Histamine is an important chemical that is needed for the efficient functioning of many body systems, particularly the brain, the digestive tract, the nervous system and the immune system. Histamine is released by the immune system when fighting foreign invaders in the body (bacteria, viruses, allergens etc.).

Excess histamine is usually broken down by enzymes in the body. However, **histamine intolerance** or sensitivity happens when an individual cannot break down histamine quickly or efficiently enough, so that they end up with more histamine in their body than is needed for normal functions. This excess of histamine can cause unpleasant symptoms.

Symptoms of Histamine Excess

These typically include[1]:

- Itching, especially of the skin, eyes, ears, and nose (known by the medical term "pruritus")
- Flushing or reddening of the skin
- Hives (known as "urticaria")
    - These are red, itchy spots or blotches on the skin that can be quite large and seem to come and go
    - Sometimes diagnosed as "idiopathic urticaria, or "autoimmune urticaria"
- Tissue swelling around the face and mouth and sometimes the throat (known by the medical term "angioedema")
    - Sometimes diagnosed as "idiopathic angioedema"
- Throat tightening

1

- Blocked nose (called "rhinitis")
- Runny nose (known by the medical term "rhinorrhea")
- Irritated, watery, reddened eyes ("conjunctivitis")
- Digestive problems, including heartburn, indigestion and reflux
- Drop in blood pressure (called "hypotension")
- Increased pulse rate
- Sensation of heart racing (also known by the medical term "tachycardia")
- Chest pain
- Symptoms resembling an anxiety or panic attack—breathing difficulties, heart racing, sweaty, feeling faint, sense of terror
- Headaches
- Psychological symptoms including confusion and irritability
- Very rarely, there may be a brief loss of consciousness usually lasting for only one or two seconds

Not all of these symptoms will occur in any one person, and the severity of symptoms will increase with the level of histamine in the body.

Nota Bene

Many of these symptoms are the same as you would suffer if you were having an allergic reaction. This is because the body releases histamine during an allergic response. Because the symptoms are so similar to allergy symptoms and are so varied, histamine intolerance is seriously under-diagnosed, even though approximately 1% of the population suffers from it[1].

Why Does Too Much Histamine Cause a Problem?

The symptoms of histamine sensitivity/intolerance only occur when there is too much histamine in the body.

Think of histamine intolerance like a bucket filling up with water. Everything is fine while the water is below the bucket's edge; however as soon as the bucket overflows, serious problems can occur. Remember too that every person has a differently-sized bucket; the point at which the bucket overflows and symptoms appear is called a person's limit of tolerance, and this limit varies between individuals.

So, why does the bucket overflow at all? Because, for various reasons, histamine levels in the body can increase to a point that at which the body can no longer cope with it.

How Does the Body Usually get Rid of Histamine?

Excess histamine is broken down and removed from the body by enzymes called DAO (diamine oxidase), and, to a lesser extent, HNMT (histamine N-methyl transferase).[2] If a person has low levels of these enzymes they will be able to tolerate less histamine—their bucket is smaller than usual!

Under normal conditions, when histamine levels rise above a certain level, these enzymes quickly break down the excess. However, when the enzymes cannot break it down fast enough, the total level of histamine in the body rises. When it reaches a critical level, it reacts with specific cells in the body and causes symptoms that are often indistinguishable from allergy.

This, obviously, happens most often in people with lower levels of histamine tolerance. However, even people who produce normal levels of the enzymes can suffer symptoms (such as severe headaches and flushing)[3] if they consume more histamine than their systems can process (i.e. by eating a meal containing massive amounts of histamine). Even a large bucket can be overfilled!

Where is Histamine Found in the Body?

In humans, the highest histamine concentrations are found in the skin, lungs, and stomach, with smaller amounts in the brain and heart. However, this is not the only source of histamine in our bodies: it is also found in the digestive tract, and released from white blood cells.

Why do Histamine Levels Increase?

It is thought that the level of histamine-regulating enzymes, especially DAO, that a person produces may be an inherited trait. It is not uncommon to see histamine intolerance running in families.

However, several diseases, conditions and hormone changes can affect histamine tolerance levels—the size of your bucket—such as:

Inflammation and allergy

When the immune system is triggered—when it is defending the body from injury or infection, or as the result of an allergic reaction— the first thing it does is release histamine, in a process called inflammation. White blood cells and proteins are stimulated, antibodies are released, and this leads to the release of defense chemicals including histamine.

Think what happens when, for example, you scratch or scrape your skin. The injury site becomes hot, reddened, sore and swollen as a result of the action of the defense chemicals, particularly histamine. This can happen anywhere in the body, but, when the injury is internal, the outward signs may be hidden but the effects are felt in various tissues and organs of the body.

Allergy is essentially an inflammatory reaction; histamine (together with other defense chemicals) is released when you come into contact with an allergen. Allergens include plant pollens, animal dander, mold spores, dust, insect stings and foods, among others. An allergic reaction occurs when the immune system mistakes these foreign (but harmless) substances for a threat.

Mastocytosis and MCAD (mast cell activation disorder)

These are conditions where excessive numbers of mast cells (a type of white blood cell called leukocytes) accumulate in various tissues, especially the skin, bone marrow, gastrointestinal tract, liver, spleen and lymph nodes.[4, 5]

This means that if someone with the condition is injured—or if anything else happens to them to trigger an inflammatory response—then histamine and the other defense chemicals are released in massive amounts from these mast cells. When this happens, the sufferer experiences all the symptoms of excess histamine.

There is more information on Mastocytosis/MCADs, including a discussion of managing the symptoms of histamine excess, later in the book.

Hormone changes

Histamine levels can be affected by hormone changes. In women, this can happen at their first menstrual period ("the menarche"), during certain phases of the menstrual cycle, and at menopause. In contrast, during pregnancy, the placenta makes a large amount of the enzyme that breaks down histamine (DAO)[6], and women cease to be sensitive to histamine during their pregnancy. However, this is only temporary, and they will become sensitive again after the child is born and the placenta is no longer available.

Men may suffer from lowered testosterone levels and an increase in progesterone, which again can heighten sensitivity to histamine.

Medical agents and medicines

Some medications and medical agents (including radiographic dyes and some agents used as part of anesthesia) release histamine, and others can reduce the effectiveness of the enzyme DAO; this means that even people who have never been sensitive to histamine in the past can suffer symptoms.

Medications that can affect histamine sensitivity:

- Some antibiotics
- Some antidepressants
- Aspirin
- Some diuretics (water pills)
- NSAIDs (nonsteroidal anti-inflammatory drugs)

If you take *any* medicine regularly, you should perform a review with your doctor to see if it is potentially influencing your histamine intolerance. SIGHI have a useful list of agents that affect histamine sensitivity, and the medications that they typically appear in[7], you may wish to discuss this with your doctor.

Diet

Certain foods can contain high levels of histamine, often as a result of manufacturing processes. Some foods and drinks (especially those containing artificial colors such as tartrazine or other azo dyes, and preservatives such as benzoates and sulfites) can also increase the amount of histamine released into the body.

The histamine-restricted diet (later in this book) covers which foods are safe to eat, and which should be avoided.

How Much Histamine is Too Much?

This varies between individuals. Histamine levels of 0.3 to 1.0 nanograms per milliliter (ng/mL) in the blood are considered to be normal[8]. However, as previously mentioned, everyone has a different tolerance threshold (i.e. their bucket size). In sensitive people, this limit will be lower than normal, and exceeding this can result in symptoms.

As histamine levels rise, the symptoms will get more severe.

How is Histamine Intolerance Diagnosed?

The short answer is, it isn't.

Histamine intolerance isn't a diagnosis in itself, because histamine excess could be the result of many different conditions and diseases. It is therefore important to consult a medical professional first, to find out whether an underlying medical condition could be causing high levels of histamine in the body.

Some practitioners offer tests to determine enzyme (DAO) levels.

_____ will not be helpful as discovering that you have low levels of DAO alone will not help anyone diagnose why you are suffering from excess histamine.

Measuring levels of histamine in your body doesn't help either, as histamine levels fluctuate throughout the day in response to need. For example, histamine levels rise after every meal because it is needed for the release of gastric acid in the stomach; this is essential for proper digestion, especially of protein.

Once a doctor has ruled out any other conditions, you can assume that you are histamine-sensitive if:

- You suffer symptoms which resemble allergic symptoms but you do not have a diagnosed allergy
- You have had skin and blood tests for specific allergies and they have been negative, suggesting that you do not have that allergy
- You have been tested for, and do not have, mastocytosis/mast cell activation disorders (MCADs)
- You do not have an autoimmune disease that could cause a chronic release of histamine
- Your symptoms improved when you spent a minimum of two weeks on the histamine-restricted diet

How can you distinguish between Histamine Intolerance and Food Allergy?

Food allergy is a hypersensitivity reaction of the immune system; when a person eats even the smallest amount of a food that they're sensitive to, defense chemicals are immediately released. Reactions to food allergies are quick, and symptoms typically appear within minutes of the food entering the body.

The same symptoms are often seen in allergic reactions and in histamine intolerance. The only difference is that it takes the symptoms much longer to appear after you have eaten histamine-rich foods or drinks, than if you had eaten a food to which you were allergic. This is because the level of histamine in your body needs to reach a critical level—your bucket needs to overflow—before your tissues respond. So, a small amount of histamine will not cause any symptoms. It is the total amount of histamine in the body, over and above what it actually needs, that causes the reaction.

Therefore, tests designed to measure an allergic reaction will not work for histamine intolerance. Symptoms will often only appear several hours after you have eaten histamine-rich foods, as the total level of histamine in your body gradually rises and overwhelms the enzymes' capacities to break it down. Meanwhile, you may have eaten a whole range of different foods, so it is almost impossible directly associate any one food with the rise in your histamine levels, and therefore your histamine intolerance.

Where Does Histamine Come from in Food?

Histamine is also to be found in the food we eat:

- Histamine is produced during the ripening of some plant foods
- Histamine is produced when fish and shellfish are not processed correctly
- Histamine occurs in some foods (like cheese, alcohol and salami) as a result of their manufacturing processes
- Histamine is released by natural and artificial chemicals
- Research is continuing into how a food such as egg white releases histamine in the body

Histamine in the ripening of fruits

Certain foods seem to contain high levels of histamine, and some studies suggest that histamine may be produced in some plants, such as tomatoes, during the ripening process. Green tomatoes contain virtually no histamine and can be eaten on the histamine-restricted diet, while red tomatoes contain a significant amount of histamine and must be avoided.

It is possible that other fruits that go through a similar process and produce histamine in the course of ripening; ripe red cherries, for example, contain more histamine than the unripe fruit. Similarly, over-ripe and rotting fruits and vegetables will be high in histamine.

Histamine caused by incorrect processing of fish or shellfish

Many reactions to fish or shellfish have been blamed on allergy, when in reality it was a reaction to an exceedingly high level of histamine in a fish that had not been processed correctly.

The guts of fish contain bacteria that produces an enzyme called histidine decarboxylase, which converts histidine to histamine. Live fish do not contain histamine, but as soon as a fish dies, its gut bacteria start to break down the tissue proteins. Histidine is released as the tissues degrade, and is rapidly converted to histamine. Since bacteria multiply extremely quickly, the level of histamine in the ungutted fish can double every twenty minutes. The longer the wait until a dead fish is gutted, the higher the level of histamine in its tissues. Also, be aware that as shellfish are not gutted after harvesting, the bacteria in their gut will keep producing histamine until they are cooked.

Histamine in manufactured foods

When food is fermented, relatively high levels of amines are produced; amines are a group of chemical compounds, including histamine. This means that any food produced with fermentation contains substantial amounts of histamine, for example:

- cheese (all types)
- alcoholic beverages
- vinegar
- fermented vegetables such as sauerkraut
- fermented soy products such as soy sauce
- processed meats such as pepperoni, bologna, salami, and frankfurters (and be aware that some sausages are also fermented, again increasing their histamine content)

There is a full list of foods to avoid, later in the book, in the section on the histamine-restricted diet.

Histamine release by natural and artificial chemicals

Research suggests that azo food dyes—such as tartrazine—and preservatives—such as benzoates and sulfites—release histamine, although we do not yet understand how.

Studies have shown that if you are sensitive to these chemicals the levels of histamine in your blood will remain high long after histamine levels in a non-sensitive person have returned to normal.

Foods that contain natural sources of these chemicals, especially benzoates, may release histamine when they are eaten. Many berries (such as strawberries, raspberries, and cranberries), vegetables (such as pumpkin and eggplant/aubergine), spices, (particularly cinnamon) and green and black tea, contain significant levels of benzoates and can contribute to the level of histamine in the body when eaten in large quantities.

Histamine derived from foods by unknown mechanisms

Traditionally, certain foods have been said to have histamine-releasing properties because when you eat them you tend to suffer from the symptoms of excess histamine. Egg white is thought to be histamine releasing—quite apart from being an allergen—although it is not known how it releases histamine.

CHAPTER 2: MANAGING HISTAMINE INTOLERANCE

The first step in managing histamine sensitivity is to discover whether there is an underlying cause for your excess histamine. Conditions mentioned above (allergy, mast cell activation disorder, autoimmune processes, infection, chronic inflammation) result in excess histamine. If you are found to have any of these and if they are treated appropriately, the symptoms of histamine excess should disappear.

This means that you should always consult a medical professional first, to ensure that your histamine excess is not due to another underlying condition that might be treated more appropriately. The advice given in this book is not a substitute for a consultation with your own doctor.

If no underlying cause can be found, then histamine intolerance should certainly be suspected and controlling the amount of histamine entering the body is generally very effective. A histamine-restricted diet combined with DAO supplements (the enzyme that breaks down excess histamine) will usually reduce histamine to a point at which you will not suffer any symptoms.

If your symptoms resolve on a histamine-restricted diet, I would recommend that you continue that regimen, but making sure that you are eating a balanced and nutritious diet from the allowed food in the list. As long as you continue the histamine restricted diet, you should not suffer any symptoms of histamine sensitivity.

Is There a Cure for This Illness or is it for Life?

The only cure for histamine intolerance is to find the cause of the excess histamine and treat it. If the underlying cause is found to be a DAO deficiency then a histamine-restricted diet, plus DAO supplements, should ensure that you remain relatively symptom-free.

However, it is important to understand that there are many different reasons for a person to have an excess of histamine in their body and all these should be investigated before deciding that DAO deficiency is the cause. When histamine in the body comes from a condition (such as mastocytosis or allergy), it will only be controlled by diagnosing and treating the underlying cause.

Histamine levels will also fluctuate with changes in hormones (especially in estrogen and progesterone levels), so the first menstrual cycle and the menopause can pose a problem for some women with histamine sensitivity.

Stress is also an important factor in histamine release and control, so look at the level of stress in your life during the times that your symptoms seem to worsen to see whether this could be a factor in any fluctuations.

Finally, please be reassured that although the symptoms can be very distressing, histamine intolerance *on its own* is not life-threatening and will not result in any permanent damage to the body. The symptoms are a result of histamine overload when the levels of histamine in the body overwhelm the enzymes' capacity to break down the excess quickly enough. When the excess histamine is finally removed from the body, the symptoms resolve and things return to normal.

How can Diet Help in Reducing Excess Histamine?

It is often difficult for people to understand that *no one food* will trigger the symptoms of histamine intolerance. Remember that it is like a bucket filling up with water. When the total level reaches the top of the bucket, the water overflows; that's the point at which symptoms appear. And histamine builds up over a long time; so, an intolerant person may not experience any symptoms for several hours after eating high-histamine foods.

Also, eating a specific food does not always result in symptoms (unlike food allergy). So, it is not possible to just avoid the foods that cause a reaction. Instead, you need to reduce the total number of high-histamine foods that you eat so that your total consumption remains below your personal limit of tolerance—and your bucket does not overflow.

However, because the total amount of histamine in the body comes from sources both inside and outside the body, simply avoiding foods with high levels of histamine will not prevent the symptoms if your bucket is already being filled up from other sources.

Symptoms of histamine excess vary for most sufferers because of outside factors. For example, if they are allergic to pollen, the histamine released in their allergic response to the pollen might already put them into a histamine overload situation. This means that their bucket will already be overflowing, so avoiding high histamine foods will not be enough to stop them from having symptoms. Many people, during their pollen allergy season, find themselves reacting to foods (usually histamine-rich foods) that they could normally eat without any problems, because their bucket is already full.

There are many factors that contribute to excess histamine, and each person's capacity to deal with it is different; this means the symptoms can change constantly both in terms of frequency and severity.

So, if someone with histamine intolerance wants to remain symptom-free, they will usually need to follow the histamine-restricted diet (featured later in this book) for the long-term. They might also benefit from taking a supplement or antihistamine—see below.

The Role of Supplements, Probiotics and Antihistamines in Treating Histamine Intolerance

Diamine Oxidase (DAO)

Under normal conditions, excess histamine is broken down by specific enzymes, especially diamine oxidase (DAO). Usually this will ensure that histamine levels do not exceed a person's limit of tolerance (i.e. their bucket does not overflow). However, when the amount of DAO is insufficient to deal with the excess, histamine levels rise and histamine sensitivity symptoms develop.

If the issue is an excess of histamine rather than an allergy to it, DAO supplements may be helpful when the diet alone cannot control symptoms. DAO supplements are designed to increase the DAO in the digestive tract and improve the breakdown of histamine in food in the digestive canal. This may reduce the body's total levels of histamine to below the person's limit of tolerance and provide relief from symptoms.

DAO must be taken immediately before meals, as it is only active for a short time. The enzyme is mixed with the food in the digestive tract and breaks down the histamine within the food so that it will not be absorbed by the body. (The DAO itself is not absorbed into the body either so it has no adverse effects.) Unlike supplements of vitamins, minerals and other nutrients, DAO does not enter the circulation and therefore will not increase the amount of DAO inside the body.

Nota Bene

To reduce your histamine level from whatever cause, you will need to follow a histamine-restricted diet *as well as* taking DAO. You cannot reduce your histamine level by simply taking DAO supplements while still consuming a diet that is high in histamine-containing foods and drinks.

FAQs about DAO

"Will DAO supplements cure me of histamine intolerance?"

No. DAO supplements reduce the amount of histamine entering the body, meaning that the total level of histamine within the body (from inside and outside sources) may then fall below your level of tolerance; this will provide relief from symptoms. However, symptoms will still develop in the future when your total level of histamine (from both internal and external sources) exceeds your limit of tolerance.

"Will taking DAO supplements regularly increase my DAO?"

No. DAO from supplements does not enter the body, so cannot increase your internal DAO. Taking the supplement regularly will only affect the amount of histamine in the food and drinks you eat or drink immediately after taking it.

"What side-effects can I expect from DAO supplements?"

Because DAO is not absorbed into the body, the DAO enzyme itself will not have any harmful effects. Any bad reactions you may have to the supplement will be due to its other ingredients that have been absorbed into the body. If you have concerns about these additives, be careful to read the list of ingredients on the product label, or ask the manufacturer for more information; obviously do not take a supplement if it contains anything to which you know you are intolerant or allergic.

"What DAO supplements are available?"

In previous years, there were a number of different DAO supplements on the market. However, at the time of writing, there is only one food-grade DAO supplement available: Umbrellux DAO (available directly from the manufacturer at www.umbrelluxdao.com).

Antihistamines

For acute episodes, when the symptoms are overwhelming, a fast-acting antihistamine such as Benadryl will be helpful. This has a sedating effect, so be aware that you will feel sleepy after taking it, and act accordingly. Antihistamines, however, do not stop the release of histamine from mast cells, so if the bucket was full before, it will still be full after taking the antihistamine, and symptoms will reoccur as soon as its effects wear off.

While antihistamines are useful for managing symptoms when they are overwhelming, taking them is not a substitute for following the histamine-restricted diet.

Stomach Acid Inhibitors

Excess histamine can trigger the release of excess gastric acid, resulting in symptoms including heartburn, indigestion and abdominal pain. There are various medications that reduce surplus stomach acid, and these can be separated into two groups:

- H2 blockers, including cimetidine and ranitidine. They work by "blocking" the histamine, thus reducing the acid production.
- Proton Pump Inhibitors (PPIs), including omeprazole and lansoprazole. They don't stop the histamine producing the acid, but instead stop acid being pumped into the stomach.

Consult your doctor to talk about your symptoms, and to discuss which of these medications may be right for you. If you suffer with gastric problems only because of excess histamine, then an H2 blocker should be enough to prevent these symptoms. PPIs are very powerful drugs, so H2 blockers are regarded as a more "natural" option.

Other supplements

Quercetin

Quercetin is often suggested as a supplement to antihistamine therapy; it is a compound (known as a bioflavonoid) found in several fruits and vegetables. It is an antioxidant and reports suggest that it stabilizes mast cells. However, if inflammation is not involved in an individual case, then it probably would have very little effect in improving symptoms.

Vitamin C
While vitamin C has antihistaminic properties, there is some evidence that vitamin C might reduce DAO activity slightly under

some conditions. So, if DAO deficiency is the cause of histamine intolerance, then you should not take large amounts of vitamin C.

Probiotics

We do know that certain strains of microorganisms produce histidine decarboxylase (which is the enzyme that converts histidine to histamine). When these strains are present in the bowel, they act on protein from undigested food in the digested tract, producing histamine that is absorbed into the body; this increases a person's total histamine level.

Presently, there is no way to specifically remove these strains from the bowel. However, we also know that some strains of microorganisms produce DAO and therefore might have the ability to break down histamine in the digestive tract, helping to reduce a person's total body level of histamine. However, again, we do not currently have any way of delivering these specific microorganisms to the digestive tract in the form of a probiotic.

Indiscriminately taking a probiotic as a treatment for histamine excess would carry the risk of actually increasing histamine if one or more of the probiotic strains produce histidine decarboxylase.

Until we know a lot more about these microorganisms, and can select individual strains successfully, it is unwise to take a probiotic in an attempt to manage histamine intolerance or sensitivity.

Zeolites

There are some claims that the zeolite clinoptilolite (a type of mineral) can help absorb and remove excess histamine. However, the value of these claims has not been proven. I would strongly urge you to consult your family doctor before embarking on a course of treatment with clinoptilolite.

In conclusion: it is very important for anyone contemplating taking supplements to understand how each supplement acts in the body and to take only those necessary to balance a deficiency. Often the consumer is unaware of detrimental effects of taking unnecessary supplements that could actually cause harm by creating an imbalance.

The Histamine-Restricted Diet: Foods to Eat, Foods to Avoid

Currently, the most effective method of reducing the symptoms of histamine intolerance is to carefully follow a histamine-restricted diet, in combination with a DAO supplement.

It's important to eat a balanced diet, and the following information will help you make informed choices.

How to follow the diet

Remember to consult your doctor before you embark on any new diet.

When following the histamine-restricted diet, it is a good idea to consult a registered dietitian. Anyone following a diet that restricts important nutrients must substitute foods of equal nutritional value to those restricted. If you are concerned that a child has histamine intolerance, you should consult a medical professional before you change their diet.

To start, follow this diet for a period of two to four weeks. If your symptoms improve you may assume that histamine sensitivity, possibly due to low DAO activity, is at least part of your problem. You will be able to control your symptoms for the long term by continuing with this diet.

While on this diet, you must make sure that you are still getting a good balance of nutritious foods. Make sure you are substituting foods of equal nutritional value to the foods that you are omitting from your diet. Eat plenty of the foods allowed while avoiding those that are not.

Long-term, you will learn more about your personal limit of

tolerance—your bucket size. As long as you do not mind the temporary return of your symptoms, then you can eat off-diet occasionally; just be sure to monitor your reaction. There will be no long-term impact on your health if you occasionally eat a 'food to avoid'.

If your symptoms do not improve during the trial period, then you can assume that you do not have a histamine intolerance, and you can go back to eating whatever you like.

General rules, hints and tips for the histamine-restricted diet

- ALWAYS READ LABELS AND CHECK INGREDIENTS LISTS. If a product contains **any** of the ingredients on the "Avoid" lists, you should not eat it.
- Freeze leftover protein foods (such as meat, poultry and fish); this slows bacterial growth (and histamine production) dramatically. Avoid eating leftover protein food that has been stored at room temperature or even in the fridge. Bacteria multiply rapidly—most strains double every 20 minutes at body temperature—and histamine content rises.
- Peel and prepare your own fruit and vegetables where possible, as close to eating as you can. Whole fresh fruits and vegetables are protected (by their peels or skins) from germs, and therefore histamine production. Pre-prepared salads, vegetables and fruit often have a higher histamine content.
- Grow your own sprouts where possible. They'll contain half the histamine of prepackaged mung bean and radish sprouts.
- Avoid foods that have been fermented by microorganisms (e.g. kefir, kombucha, sauerkraut). The fermentation process can lead to high histamine levels.

- Beware food additives as they can release histamine. This includes artificial colors such as FD&C Yellow #5 (tartrazine) and preservatives such as benzoates and sulfites; these are also sometimes found in medications.
- Ensure any medications or supplements that you take are free from artificial colors and preservatives; ask your doctor or pharmacist for more information.
- Vitamin B3 (Niacin) can cause issues for histamine intolerance sufferers. Avoid any supplements that contain niacin and look for products containing niacinamide instead.
- Read the labels on your toiletries carefully and avoid any products that contain cinnamaldehyde, balsam of Peru, benzoates of any kind, sulfites and FD&C Yellow #5 (tartrazine). These substances may cause skin rash.

Safe to eat, foods to avoid: what to eat on the histamine-restricted diet

Please remember to check the ingredients list carefully on everything you buy; if a product contains **any** of the ingredients on the Avoid list, you should not eat it. Make sure that you eat a good variety of the allowed foods to ensure a complete balance of nutrition.

Meat & poultry

Safe to eat

- All types of plain, freshly cooked meat or poultry (e.g. beef, pork, lamb, venison, moose, elk, chicken, turkey, goose, ostrich, duck, pheasant, etc.)
- Freeze dried meat

Avoid

- All leftover cooked meat, unless frozen immediately and reheated before consumption.
- Processed, smoked, pickled or fermented meats such as luncheon meat, sausage, wiener, hot dogs, bologna, salami, pepperoni, smoked ham, cured bacon and Parma ham.

Fish

Safe to eat

- Fish that has been caught, gutted and cooked within thirty minutes (it should not smell fishy—beware fish that does, as this usually means that there has been a lot of microbial activity).
- Fish that has been frozen or canned in North America or the EU.

Avoid

- All shellfish unless you can ensure that they are cooked from the live state
- Any fish—whether fresh, frozen, smoked or canned/tinned—if you do not know how it has been processed.
- Pickled fish
- Smoked fish (e.g. smoked salmon; smoked trout)

Egg

Egg whites release histamine by a mechanism that we do not

understand, whereas egg yolks are usually safe. Whole eggs are OK as a minor ingredient, however do check the list below:

Safe to eat

- A small quantity of cooked egg in baked products (such as pancakes, muffins and cakes) is allowed.
  - Typically, a slice of cake contains around a quarter of an egg, which is OK.

Avoid

- Dishes containing raw egg. For example:
  - Eggnog
  - Hollandaise sauce
  - Salad dressing (such as Caesar dressing)
- Eggs as a feature in their own right
  - Including fried, hard-cooked/hard-boiled, poached and scrambled eggs.
- Mayonnaise (both homemade and commercially produced)
- Any dish where eggs are the main ingredient. For example:
  - Custard
  - Meringue
  - Mousse
  - Omelet/omelette
  - Pavlova
  - Quiche
  - Soufflé

Milk and dairy

Safe to eat

- Cream
- Curdled milk products (including panir/paneer)

- o as long as they have been produced without microbial fermentation (check labels for words like "bacterial culture" or "microbial culture"; any foods that suggest microorganisms in their ingredients should be avoided)
- Ice cream
  - o as long as it is free from artificial additives (e.g. preservatives, emulsion factors, artificial colors, artificial flavors).
- Milk is an excellent source of protein.
  - o Choose plain milk, including whole, reduced-fat (2%), semi-skimmed, low-fat (1%), and fat-free (skim/skimmed)
  - o All animal milk is safe (e.g. cow, goat, sheep)

Avoid

All *fermented* milk products, including:

- Buttermilk
- Cheese made by fermentation (e.g. cheddar, blue cheese, brie)
- Cheese products: processed cheese, cheese slices, cheese spreads
- Cottage cheese
- Kefir, and other milk products produced by fermentation
- Ricotta (if made with bacterial culture)
- Sour/soured cream, also crème fraiche
- Yoghurt

Grains and starches
(including rice, pasta, sweet products, bread products and cereal)

Safe to eat

A quick reminder to check ingredient lists in everything you buy; do not consume anything that contains ingredients from any of the "Avoid" lists.

- Bread, buns and biscuits (US)
  - Choose plain, fresh whole grain products
- Cakes, cookies (US)/biscuits (UK) and pies
- Cereal
  - Choose plain grain breakfast cereals such as: Cornflakes, Shredded Wheat, Rice Krispies, plain oats, oatmeal, cream of wheat, puffed wheat, puffed rice, and cream of rice
- Corn, cornstarch, cornmeal and cornflour
- Crackers
  - Choose plain crackers such as Grissol Melba Toast, Ryvita, Rye Krisp, Wassa Crisp Bread, rice cakes and rice crackers
- Oats
- Pasta (plain)
- Pastries (homemade)
- Pizza dough
- Popcorn (plain)
- Rice
  - All types of rice are fine—including instant or parboiled rice—as long as it is plain.
- White flour (unbleached)
- Whole grains (plain)

- Bleached flour (benzoyl peroxide is likely to be the bleaching agent)
- Cereals with artificial colors, flavors, preservatives, etc.
    - o Also avoid flavored instant oatmeal
- Pasta meals in packages or cans
- Pastries (commercially made)
- Popcorn with artificial flavors
- Rice entrees in packages or cans

Fruit

If you are buying dried fruits, avoid any that contain sulfites.

Safe to eat

- Apples
- Bananas
- Blueberries (see note at the end of this section, as blueberries may cause problems for the most histamine-sensitive people)
- Dragon Fruit
- Figs
- Guavas
- Kiwis
- Longans
- Lychees/Lichis
- Mangos
- Melons
    - o All types, e.g. cantaloupe, honeydew and watermelon
- Passion fruits
- Peaches
- Pears

Rhubarb
- Starfruits

- Apricots
- Cherries
- Cranberries
- Currants
- Dates
- Grapefruit
- Grapes
- Lemons
- Limes
- Loganberries
- Mulberries
- Nectarines
- Oranges
- Papayas/Pawpaws
- Pineapple
- Plums
- Prunes
- Raisins
- Raspberries
- Saskatoon berries
- Strawberries

Vegetables

Safe to eat

All plain vegetables—whether fresh, frozen, canned, juiced—except for those on the "Avoid" list. This also includes leaves like kale and arugula/rocket, but not spinach.

Avoid

- Avocado
- Eggplant/aubergine
- Olives
- Pumpkin
- Ripe Tomatoes (including tomato sauces & ketchup)
  - Green, unripe tomatoes are OK
- Spinach

Legumes

(Beans, Lentils, Peanuts, Peas)

Safe to eat

- All fresh, frozen, canned/tinned beans and peas (except those on the "Avoid" list)
- Peanuts
- Plain peanut butter

Avoid

- Garbanzo beans/chick peas
- Lentils
- Red beans (such as kidney beans and adzuki beans)
- Soybeans/edamame
- Soy products; this includes
  - Miso
  - Soy lecithin/soya lecithin
  - Soy milk/Soya milk
  - Soy sauce/Soya sauce
  - Tofu

Nuts and seeds

Safe to eat

All plain nuts and seeds (excluding pumpkin seeds)

Avoid

- Nut and seed mixtures with artificial flavoring (such as barbecue, chilli, ranch)
- Pumpkin seeds

Herbs, spices and seasonings

Safe to eat

- All plain fresh, frozen or dried herbs (except for those on the "Avoid" list)
- All plain spices (except for those on the "Avoid" list)

Avoid

- Anise
- Chili powder (commercial mixes usually contain restricted spices)
- Cinnamon
- Cloves
- Commercial mixes/seasoning packages which contain restricted spices
- Curry powder (commercial mixes usually contain restricted spices)
- Foods labelled "…with spices"

- Nutmeg
- Thyme

Fats and oils

Safe to eat

- Butter (plain)
- Gravy (homemade)
- Lard and meat drippings/dripping
- Pure vegetable oil, *except* olive oil
- Salad dressing (homemade with allowed ingredients)

Avoid

- Any fats and oils with added color and/or preservatives
- Gravy made from mixes, or from cans
- Hydrolysed/hydrolyzed lecithin
- Margarine
- Olive oil

Candies, sugar and sweeteners

Safe to eat

- Corn syrup
- Candies/sweets (homemade with allowed ingredients)
- Honey
- Jams, jellies, marmalades and preserves (made with allowed ingredients)
- Maple syrup

- Plain artificial sweeteners
- Sugar (all kinds)

Avoid

- Cake decorations
- Chocolate
- Commercial candies/sweets
- Commercial frosting
- Commercial prepared dessert fillings
- Flavored syrups

Drinks/beverages

Safe to drink

- 100% fruit and vegetable juices (from "Safe to Eat" ingredients)
- Coffee (plain)
- Cocoa (homemade with allowed ingredients: baking cocoa is allowed)
- Herbal teas
    - Check ingredients, and avoid spices (no "Zingers" or "Zests")
- Milk (plain)
- Mineral Water (plain)
    - Still and carbonated

Avoid

- All alcoholic drinks
- All "flavored" drinks
- Cola-type carbonated drinks; "sodas"

- Fermented drinks (e.g. kombucha, kefir)
- Flavored coffees
- Flavored milks
- Non-alcoholic beers/wines and other beverages from which the alcohol has been removed but have been produced by fermentation
- Tea
  o Regular and green

Miscellaneous

Safe to eat

- Baking powder
- Baking soda
- Cornstarch/cornflour
- Cream of tartar
- Fish oil
- Gelatin (plain)
- Homemade relish (made from "Safe to Eat" ingredients)
- Yeast

Avoid

- Artificial colors (e.g. tartrazine)
- Fermented food (e.g. sauerkraut)
- Flavored gelatin
- Tomato ketchup
- Medicines and vitamin pills containing artificial colors, benzoates or sulfites
- Mincemeat (i.e. mixed chopped dried fruit, with spices and spirits)
- Pickles
- Relish (pre-prepared)
- Preservatives, especially benzoates and sulfites

- Soy and soy products (see "Legumes" section above for more information)
- Vinegar

Questions related to the histamine-restricted diet, and other diet programs

Berries

Question:

"Why are blueberries on safe to eat when other types of berries aren't?"

Dr. Joneja replies:

Berries tend to contain varying levels of benzoates that trigger the release of histamine in certain people. The highest levels of benzoates in berries are found in strawberries, raspberries and cranberries. Blueberries have very little benzoate so are probably safe for most histamine-sensitive people; proceed with caution, however, if you are particularly sensitive as you may need to exclude blueberries from your diet.

Mastocytosis/Mast cell activation disorders

Question:

"If the cause of histamine intolerance or excess histamine is a mast cell disorder (like mast cell activation syndrome), and not DAO deficiency, would a low-histamine diet help to reduce symptoms? Or should people with mast cell disorders only stay away from foods that are histamine liberators, like strawberries and egg white?"

Dr. Joneja Replies:

Mast cell activation disorders involve an overabundance of defense chemicals, including histamine. A histamine-restricted diet will reduce the effects of the excess histamine in mast cell activation disorders, but will have little effect in counteracting the other mediators.

Simply avoiding foods such as strawberries and egg whites will not have any noticeable effect on either histamine sensitivity as a result of DAO deficiency, or excess histamine released in mast cell activation disorders. In either situation, it is necessary to avoid *all* histamine-associated foods (i.e. histamine-containing, and histamine-releasing foods and additives) to reduce the histamine level below a person's limit of tolerance.

Protein

Question:

'My physician says that I need to eat a little protein at every meal. Would protein powders containing rice or pea protein be safe?'

Dr. Joneja replies:

The histamine-restricted diet provides you with a comprehensive list of protein foods. I do not recommend supplements such as protein powders for nutrients that you can obtain from natural foods because all supplements, being manufactured products, will contain various additives that a food-sensitive person needs to avoid.

Reoccurrence of symptoms while following the histamine-restricted diet

Question:

"I am a 16-year-old female and have been recently diagnosed with histamine intolerance by my dietitian. My symptoms include daily headaches and migraines, fatigue, dizziness, stomach cramps, chest pain, brain fog and poor concentration, nausea, tingling in my hands and feet, shortness of breath, poor balance, sour-smelling urine and non-epileptic seizures caused by anxiety and stress.

I have been on a low histamine diet for about two months, and I felt so much better for the first few weeks. My headaches decreased dramatically, I felt less sluggish, I could concentrate a bit better and my other symptoms decreased. However, in the last three weeks, I haven't been feeling great and my symptoms have been returning while I am still on the low histamine diet. Why is this? Am I not getting enough nutrients from my diet? I have been trying to include a wide variety of foods in my low-histamine diet. Is there something else going on? Should I consider mastocytosis?"

Dr. Joneja replies:

The symptoms you list might indicate several different disorders and it is very important that investigations be undertaken by your doctors to determine any underlying causes. Histamine excess can result from many different illnesses. Any condition that results in histamine release within the body, such as infection, inflammation, autoimmune conditions and allergy, among others, can cause a build-up of histamine that exceeds the ability of the enzymes to break it down fast enough. Furthermore, anxiety and stress can make the situation worse by increasing the quantity of histamine released.

It is possible that the histamine-restricted diet improved your symptoms by reducing the amount of histamine coming from outside sources—that is, your diet. However, if the histamine is arising inside your body from any of the causes I have suggested, the histamine-restricted diet alone will be insufficient to keep your histamine levels below your limit of tolerance—that is, below the level at which symptoms develop. The diet will only help to decrease the top layer of histamine filling up the bucket; the underlying condition will cause the level to rise near, or over the top of the bucket, where the enzymes are overwhelmed and unable to efficiently remove the excess to keep you symptom-free. Histamine from internal sources can fluctuate quite significantly, so sometimes the diet will help, at other times it will not reduce your histamine level sufficiently to relieve your symptoms.

It would be a good idea for your doctors to investigate the possibility that you might have some form of mast cell activation disorder (MCAD/mastocytosis). Too many mast cells most certainly would result in excess histamine when conditions trigger the release of the inflammatory mediators, which include histamine, stored within. There are several tests available for diagnosis of mastocytosis, and I would encourage you to discuss this with your doctors as soon as possible.

Rotation Diets

Question:

"My MD told me to adhere to a rotation diet so I don't become sensitized to more foods. How does this work with the histamine-restricted diet?"

Dr. Joneja replies:

A rotation diet is a plan of eating that is based around "food families". These are biologically-related foods: for example, the Nightshade food family includes eggplant/aubergine, bell peppers, tomato and potatoes, amongst others. So, biologically-related foods are eaten on the same day, and then not eaten again for four days. However, most authorities consider rotation diets, as a management strategy for food allergy and intolerance, to be controversial and of little or no benefit. Because cross-reactivity between foods within a food family is unusual, diets that are based on the avoidance of entire food families are illogical. Furthermore, following a strict rotation diet can be tedious and time-consuming and can cause unnecessary risk of nutritional deficiency.

Rotation Diets and Food Allergy

Eating the same food repeatedly is most unlikely to lead to sensitization, whereas avoidance of a food for a long period frequently results in loss of tolerance to it. When the person tries to eat a food after a long period of eliminating it from their diet they often have an adverse reaction to it.

Rotation Diets and Food Intolerance

When you react badly to a food ingredient but this is not an allergic reaction (one involving your immune system), limiting the amount you eat of that food or ingredient makes sense. Where you have an enzyme deficiency, such as, for example, lack of lactase, consuming a greater quantity of lactose than the enzyme can process will lead to the development of intolerance symptoms. A diet that restricts the intake of all lactose-containing foods will ensure that the limit of tolerance is not exceeded, and the person can remain symptom-free. A similar situation probably exists for most food intolerances, so a type of rotation diet that restricts the number and quantity of foods known to contain the culprit ingredients is necessary. Such diets need to be formulated on an individual basis to ensure that the dose of the ingredient is reduced to a minimum, while nutrients equivalent to those eliminated are supplied by alternative foods.

CHAPTER 3: OTHER CONDITIONS AND RELATED INFORMATION

Mastocytosis/Mast Cell Activation Disorder (MCADs)

MCADs (also known as MCAS, "mast cell activation syndrome") and mastocytosis are conditions based on a genetic mutation that results in the production of excessive numbers of mast cells. Mast cells are white blood cells (called "leukocytes") that are located in tissues throughout the body; other types of white blood cells tend to circulate in blood instead. There are especially large numbers of mast cells in the skin, respiratory tract, digestive tract, urinary tract, around blood vessels and lymphatic vessels, around nerves, and in reproductive organs.

Mast cells manufacture and store chemicals that are designed to protect the body from threat, such as infection, trauma, and other dangers and diseases, and to aid in the repair of tissues once the threat has been eradicated. They are also responsible for the allergic reaction, which in effect is a "protective" response to a foreign agent entering the body, albeit a misguided one.

Mast cells do not only release histamine, but are responsible for releasing many reactive agents that induce symptoms in addition to those produced by histamine. When there is an excessive number of mast cells in any organ, a vastly increased quantity of inflammatory mediators is released whenever an event triggers degranulation ("release of the granules"). This results in the distressing symptoms typically experienced by people suffering from mast cell activation disorder.

In systemic mastocytosis and mast cell activation disorders, many of the symptoms experienced, but by no means all, will be caused by histamine excess. Therefore, a histamine-restricted diet will reduce the amount of histamine in the body by limiting the amount of exogenous ("from outside the body") histamine contributing to the total. However, because the excess histamine is being released from mast cells within the body ("endogenous histamine"), a histamine-restricted diet would be expected to improve a person's symptoms, but not to eliminate them altogether. Furthermore, because inflammatory mediators in addition to histamine are released in mast cell degranulation, other symptoms for which histamine is not responsible, will not be affected.

So, while a histamine-restricted diet will help to improve the symptoms associated with histamine, because histamine is not the only culprit, symptoms caused by the other inflammatory mediators released from excessive numbers of mast cells will continue to be a problem and may need to be controlled by appropriate medications.

Diabetes

There is no scientific evidence for an association between Type I diabetes and histamine sensitivity. However, in cases where a diabetic suspects that they *also* suffer from histamine sensitivity, antihistamines would be the best method of controlling the symptoms in the first instance.

However, if after several months, the symptoms have not abated, a time-limited trial on a histamine-restricted diet will indicate if a dietary approach will manage the symptoms without the need for antihistamines. The diabetic patient would need the help of a registered dietitian to develop a diet that will avoid the histamine-associated foods and incorporate the foods allowed into a diabetic meal plan. It is not a difficult process, but does require careful planning to achieve a diet that provides all the nutrients required, in the appropriate quantities and at the times indicated by one's insulin intake, while avoiding those foods that could trigger a reaction.

Digestive Tract Issues, Diarrhea and IBS

In cases of prolonged diarrhea, a consultation with a gastroenterologist should be the first step. The specialist will look for any signs of disease or inflammation. Typically, there will be several tests and procedures, possibly including colonoscopy.

If these investigations don't reveal a cause for the patient's symptoms, the doctor will often consider irritable bowel syndrome (IBS) as the root of the problem. However, the disease remains a diagnosis of exclusion: this means that when all other reasons for the patient's symptoms have been ruled out, IBS is the usual verdict.

IBS is often referred to as a "functional gastrointestinal disorders" (FGID). This is a medical condition that impairs the normal function of a bodily process, but where every part of the body looks completely normal under examination, dissection or even under a microscope. FGIDs can be due to a number of factors, including the speed at which food passes through the digestive tract, plus psychosocial factors, such as stress, anxiety and depression. "Disturbed sensation" can also be a factor; this is where the patient's nervous system is not working correctly, leading the brain to receive incorrect messages, including an enhanced perception of pain.

When one considers all those potential triggers, it becomes

apparent that a common factor may be a process that is likely to involve increased numbers of mast cells. This leads to the release of a higher level of their stored defense chemicals, including histamine, exceeding a person's level of histamine tolerance. As a result, symptoms of histamine excess develop. Rashes, itching eyes, colic, and other symptoms of histamine intolerance would be expected.

In this case histamine is a *result*, not a *cause* of IBS or FGID. The symptoms of histamine sensitivity are a result of mast cell activation. A histamine-restricted diet will aid in alleviating the symptoms of histamine excess, but will not help the symptoms of IBS or FGID.

The important message here is that when the underlying cause for the IBS or FGID is identified and treated—usually by medications, diet, or lifestyle changes—the level of histamine will decrease and the symptoms of histamine excess will abate.

CHAPTER 4: CASE STUDIES

Anaphylaxis

Question:

"My 34-year-old daughter has severe anaphylaxis to milk protein, and Type 1 diabetes, celiac disease, and asthma. Normally her anaphylaxis is triggered immediately when she eats a food contaminated with milk protein. Over the last year, she has had three anaphylaxis episodes after eating in restaurants.

The first one happened three hours after eating lunch in a restaurant. She is quite sure she did not ingest dairy. The second one happened after brunch in a restaurant, but again hours after eating the food. That time she had eggs, potatoes and fruit as well as two alcoholic drinks. She woke up from a nap with anaphylaxis.

The third severe anaphylaxis happened during sleep, after eating shrimp ceviche and having two drinks about seven or eight hours earlier in a restaurant. She had to be taken by ambulance to the hospital. She was covered head to toe in hives, had a severe gut issue, very low blood pressure, heartburn, heart racing, etc. She has eaten at this restaurant many times but had never had the ceviche which is raw shrimp cured in lime juice. She went back to the restaurant and the manager assured her there was no dairy, but her reaction was like a delayed dairy reaction. What tests could she take to see if she is histamine intolerant?"

Dr. Joneja replies:

There are two points to consider in this case:

- Your daughter's diagnosed allergy to milk proteins, which has resulted in anaphylaxis in the past
- The delayed reaction to a meal extremely high in histamine

An allergic reaction involves release of inflammatory mediators from primed mast cells. The first powerful mediator released is histamine, followed by a number of others, each of which has its own effect in the body. The symptoms typically occur within minutes, even seconds, of the allergenic food entering the body. In an anaphylactic reaction, the symptoms are severe and in rare cases can lead to anaphylactic shock and death.

It is known that an allergic reaction can escalate to life-threatening anaphylaxis in people who also have histamine intolerance. A person with a severe allergy who consumes a diet rich in histamine-containing and releasing foods is at risk for both an enhanced allergic reaction ("anaphylaxis") and/or an exaggerated response to histamine.

In your daughter's case, each of the restaurant meals you mention are very high in histamine. Specifically, ceviche is an appetizer made from raw fish marinated in lime or lemon juice with olive oil and spices. All those ingredients are high in histamine and are not allowed on a histamine-restricted diet. Furthermore, the addition of alcoholic drinks will increase the level of histamine enormously.

This meal likely overwhelmed her DAO's ability to rid her body of excess histamine and resulted in a reaction that resulted in all the symptoms of anaphylaxis, but which were delayed, rather than immediate. This reaction was likely due to histamine rather than an anaphylactic reaction, but nevertheless it would be wise for your daughter to undergo further investigations to identify other foods in addition to milk to which she may be allergic, before concluding that the reactions were indeed due to histamine intolerance rather than allergy.

Unfortunately, as explained previously, we do not have any accurate tests that would provide a diagnosis of histamine intolerance.

My advice to your daughter, first of all, is to carry injectable adrenalin (e.g. an EpiPen or similar) for immediate use at the onset of an anaphylactic reaction. She should speak to her doctor about this as soon as possible if she does not already carry such a device. It would be wise for her to follow the histamine-restricted diet to reduce her body's histamine level on a regular basis. Because of her Type 1 diabetes your daughter should consult a registered dietitian to formulate a diet that will incorporate the histamine-restricted dietary protocols into her diabetic eating schedule. It is very important that she obtain complete balanced nutrition in spite of her dietary limitations. In addition, she should take a DAO supplement immediately before a meal likely to be high in histamine—such as in a restaurant—to reduce her risk of such severe reactions in the future.

Angioedema ("Swelling Under the Skin") and Urticaria ("Hives") After Food Poisoning

Question:

"I'm a 45-year-old woman who got food poisoning last October in Cabo, Mexico. Three weeks later, I started getting angioedema of eyes in the morning, on a weekly basis. These then morphed into hives, reddening of cheeks and itchy bumps on cheeks, mostly after I eat.

I've been clinically cleared of all diseases, but I'm convinced something went wrong after Cabo and my body can't break down histamines any more. How can I help my body go back to pre-Cabo where I ate everything?"

Dr. Joneja replies:

The symptoms you describe are the result of excess histamine, but the source of the excess could be one of several causes.

In answering your questions, I am impeded by the absence of some key facts:

- Was the cause of your food poisoning diagnosed?
- Did you receive any treatment in the form of antibiotics for the food poisoning or did you wait for it to clear up on its own?
- Do you have any allergies to inhalants such as pollens or other environmental allergens?
- Do you have any symptoms of menopause or perimenopause?

The details will affect my answers to your questions for the following reasons:

- If your food poisoning was due to an infective microorganism you may have received an oral antibiotic to treat the condition. This may have affected your normal bowel microflora which could have resulted in an increase in bacteria that are able to produce the enzyme histidine decarboxylase. This enzyme will convert histidine in undigested proteins into histamine in your digestive tract. Such histamine can increase the level of histamine in your body and result in the symptoms you describe.
- You state that you have "been clinically cleared of all diseases", so I am assuming that stool tests have not produced any evidence of an infective microorganism remaining in your digestive tract. Thus, we can assume that no new strains have been introduced as a result of the contaminated food.
- If the food poisoning was due to a toxin in the food you consumed, you would not have been given an antibiotic. The symptoms would have cleared up on their own

without treatment as your immune system would have gradually removed the toxin from your body. In this case your normal microflora would likely remain unchanged.

- We cannot assume that your excess histamine is a result of the food poisoning because there are several other reasons for your reactions, including respiratory allergies. This is the season when there is a significant increase in air-borne allergens and this year the pollen count in many areas is especially high. You report that your symptoms are noticeable just after eating. This is a fairly common observation in people who have seasonal inhalant allergies as histamine is released every time a person eats because the histamine is required for the release of gastric acid—an essential part of protein digestion. Therefore, if a person's "histamine bucket" is almost full as a result of an allergy, the increase in histamine triggered by the process of eating will cause the bucket to over-flow and result in symptoms such as you describe.

- If you are in, or reaching menopause, the levels of hormones such as estrogen and progesterone may be fluctuating. Such changes can affect the level of histamine in your body and result in symptoms due to histamine excess.

To answer your specific questions in light of this information:

- Your statement that possibly your body "can't breakdown histamines any more" is actually incorrect. The level of the enzymes that break down histamine, diamine oxidase (DAO) and histamine N-methyltransferase (HNMT) do not change. You will still be producing the same amount of each of these as you did prior to your food poisoning episode. The change in your histamine level is due to the amount of histamine in your body now exceeding the capacity of these enzymes to break down the excess fast enough to prevent the development of symptoms. You need to reduce the level of histamine in order to remain below your body's "limit of tolerance'—the level above which symptoms develop.

51

The most effective way for you to manage your excess histamine and to reduce your reliance on antihistamines is to closely follow my histamine-restricted diet for a trial period. If you find that your symptoms resolve, or diminish in intensity, you will be able to control your reactions by dietary management. Supplementary diamine oxide, taken before eating, will further help by reducing the amount of histamine in the food.

If your histamine excess is indeed due to a change in the microbial flora of your bowel ("your microbiome") and no other cause, you may find that over time you will begin to tolerate more histamine-containing and releasing foods as your microbiome returns to its normal composition.

Anxiety

Question:

"I turned 50 last September. Two years ago, one of my eyes got really itchy, and swelled hugely when I rubbed it. This has happened several times since then, but getting more severe each time; now both eyes swell up, plus I have a lot of anxiety and panic. My back and breasts also get itchy sometimes.

I have recently been hospitalized with panic attacks, and they gave me Benadryl and an EpiPen—which of course gave me more anxiety. Recently I have broken out in hives. I try not to panic now and take a Reactine right away and this has seemed to help so far.

I've been to an allergist and he has told me I have seasonal allergies to ragweed, pollen and grass, plus cocomadropyl betaine and gluteral, and cobalt, but all unequivocal, so I have tried not to have these ingredients in my toiletries. He said I don't have food allergies although my last test showed onion and rye, however I am on a very restrictive diet, in case it really is an allergic reaction, and have lost an incredible amount of weight. Does this sound like histamine intolerance to you?"

Dr. Joneja replies:

The symptoms you report and their onset presents a picture that I see often in my practice. The rather frightening appearance of what seems to be signs of a severe allergic reaction, associated with high anxiety, closely resembles an anaphylactic reaction. In most cases the sufferer rushes to the hospital fearing the worst. So often the patient is treated with a quick-acting antihistamine (usually Benadryl) the reaction subsides, and he or she is sent home, usually with an EpiPen. Subsequent consultation with an allergist typically results in negative reactions to all the common allergens and after several such episodes without a clear-cut diagnosis the suspicion of a psychosomatic cause for the repeated reactions is raised. Sometimes the patient is referred to psychiatric services for management of their panic attacks, which is frequently unsuccessful.

I first reported the association between histamine intolerance and anxiety and panic attacks in my 2001 paper, *Outcome of a histamine-restricted diet based on chart audit.* I had noticed that several of my patients with histamine intolerance reported that their "panic attacks" had completely resolved after they had carefully followed the histamine-restricted diet which I had prescribed for their symptoms of histamine intolerance. In all cases I had previously been completely unaware of the panic attacks since neither I nor they had thought to mention their occurrence during our consultation sessions. As a side note: I wonder how many people now being treated by psychiatrists and psychologists for "panic attacks" are actually experiencing histamine intolerance, and would respond well to a histamine-restricted diet?

Anxiety or feelings of panic are quite understandable when one considers the progression of a histamine sensitivity reaction. Histamine causes the widening of blood vessels as part of its mode of action. This allows more blood into the reaction site in a protective inflammatory response. As a result of the widening of the blood vessels there is less resistance to the heart pumping the blood, so blood pressure drops. This triggers a response of the cardiovascular system that increases the heart rate ("tachycardia") and causes feelings of high anxiety or panic because it appears that the body is under immediate threat. This same effect occurs during an anaphylactic reaction because a large quantity of histamine is released in that response. However excessive histamine in histamine intolerance is the only inflammatory mediator ("biochemical agent that causes or "mediates" reactions in the immune system") involved, whereas in an anaphylactic reaction, many more powerful mediators are activated, which in severe cases can result in cardiovascular collapse and death. A histamine reaction *alone* will never result in death, even without treatment, regardless of how ill the patient feels.

You report the onset of your symptoms as itching (in your eye), and swelling. The next array of symptoms included sneezing, runny nose, eye swelling, and panic. Later you report hives, and itching on your back and breasts. These symptoms are entirely typical of excess histamine. Your allergist diagnosed environmental allergies, which of course will lead to the release their own battery of inflammatory mediators, including high levels of histamine, thus contributing further to the total amount of histamine in your body.

So why, two years ago, did these symptoms suddenly appear, apparently out of the blue? The answer lies in the fact that you are now 50 years of age. Two years ago you likely entered perimenopause, or menopause, and your hormone levels, especially estrogen and progesterone, changed dramatically. As a result, the histamine controls in your body were affected, and you developed histamine intolerance. This is a relatively common observation in people who are likely to have a lower than normal level of the enzymes that break down excess histamine as it arises in the body in order to maintain a "normal" (non-reactive) level. This is usually an inherited condition, so I would not be surprised to learn that other members of your family have experienced similar reactions.

So—what can you do about this? Unfortunately, as we have seen earlier in the book, in spite of what you may now read on the internet, there are no tests for histamine intolerance at this time. The indicators for histamine intolerance are as I have described: symptoms resembling allergy in the absence of diagnosed allergy.

The condition is best managed by closely following a histamine-restricted diet, being very careful to replace all the restricted foods with "safe", allowed foods of equal nutritional value. You should never lose weight on this diet as it will provide all the macro- and micronutrients your body requires. When the diet alone is insufficient (in your case, probably during the season in which you are exposed to your environmental allergens), supplemental DAO could be helpful.

Dust Mite Allergy and Grief

Question:

"I'm a 38-year-old female. When I moved to the US, I developed an allergy to dust mites (which could largely be controlled with over-the-counter antihistamines). This coincided with my mother's death and a change in my diet (consuming orange juice, cheese and processed foods for the first time). When I moved to Singapore in 2009, my dust mite allergy got progressively worse to the extent that I could no longer sleep on mattresses; I had to give up using pillows and started sleeping on the floor! Every few months, I would develop severe allergic rhinitis.

I moved back to India in 2015 and started avoiding acidic and carbonated foods. Avoiding a lot of the foods as per the histamine-restricted diet has also helped tremendously; my dust mite allergies have nearly disappeared and my rhinitis symptoms are much less severe. I suspect I am histamine intolerant, however I haven't seen any research on the connection between histamine intolerance and dust mite allergies. Do you have any insight into this?"

Dr. Joneja replies:

In considering histamine sensitivity, it is important to determine the source of the excess histamine. Symptoms of allergy are caused by the release of inflammatory mediators from mast cells and other granulocytes. Histamine is the first of these to be released in significant amounts, so many of the symptoms of allergy are a result of its activities. Therefore, the symptoms of your dust mite allergy are a result of histamine excess in addition to those triggered by other inflammatory mediators released at the same time, or later.

If a person has a deficiency in either of the enzymes that break down histamine (DAO and, to a lesser extent, HNMT), the allergic reaction may be more severe, as the histamine released in the allergic response rises higher than normal and usually persists for a longer period of time. In some people with certain food allergies and allergies to drugs and injected allergens such as insect venom, this may put them at risk of a life-threatening anaphylactic reaction.

From your question, it would appear that you may have both an allergy to dust mites and a deficiency in DAO. This would explain your observation that a histamine-restricted diet allows you to encounter dust mites, to which you are still allergic, but not to react to them to the degree that you would when consuming a diet high in histamine containing and releasing foods. In fact, if a person who does not have a DAO deficiency consumes a histamine-restricted diet it may be sufficient for them to reduce the histamine resulting from the allergy to the level at which their symptoms are tolerable.

It is undeniable that stress will cause an increase in histamine in some people—also see the case study "Urticaria, ("Hives"), Stress and Depression" later in this section. Therefore, the stress of your mother's death could have been responsible for an increase in your histamine levels, and hence your observation that your allergies were more evident as a result.

Facial Rash, Low Energy, Burning Eyes, Anxiety Attacks, Hair Loss, Weight Loss and Poor Sleep

Question:

"I am a relatively healthy 43-year-old female who has had ongoing problems for the last year. It started with a few bumps under my right nostril resembling poison ivy, but this rash never went away. Several months later, the rash was still there, and my dermatologist gave me an oral antibiotic that made me very ill, and an antibiotic lotion that I believe I'm allergic to. I used it for a few months anyway, but the rash became worse—it spread around my mouth and chin.

A while after that, I started developing a bright red ring around my mouth—from my nostrils around my lips and chin—while eating meals. It looked as though someone had drawn a ring on my face with red lipstick. At first it disappeared within 15 minutes, and I had no feeling of it whatsoever. However, this gradually worsened over time, until having a few sips of white wine made my whole face immediately burn and tingle for 45 minutes.

My doctor told me to stop eating dairy, soy, sugar, gluten, wheat, most fruits, processed foods, condiments, etc. etc. I've been told I'm perimenopausal by one doctor, and been called crazy and told to see a psychiatrist. I've had an Organic Acid test for leaky gut syndrome—my oxalates were off the chart, and I had zero Vitamin C present. Several blood tests have been done, and the only thing that came back abnormal was my cortisol level.

I have low energy, my hair is falling out, and my body aches for no apparent reason. My eyes burn quite a bit and I can't tell you the last time I slept through the night. I've also been having frequent anxiety attacks, and I've lost 30 pounds in the last six months. Pineapple makes me itch terribly, as does wine or anything with vinegar. I take a vitamin B and C supplement and a calcium D3 supplement daily. I feel like a science experiment!! Do you think this could be a histamine intolerance?"

Dr. Joneja replies:

There is certainly strong evidence that your symptoms are mediated by histamine. Whenever there is inflammation, rash, reddening, burning, or itching, histamine is involved. However, the question is, what is the cause of the excess histamine?

You mention that you are in perimenopause, which involves a significant change in hormone levels. We know that estrogen, and especially progesterone, have a direct effect in histamine control mechanisms, so it is very likely that this is an important factor in the triggering of your symptoms.

I am alarmed that your doctor directed you to avoid a long list of foods, apparently without any evidence of their involvement in your condition. No health care provider should indiscriminately advise a patient to avoid foods without (1) Evidence of their role in the condition and (2) Provision of a diet that will supply all nutrients from alternate sources. In my practice, I see this too often and it causes me great concern as it puts the patient at risk for nutritional deficiency and tends to direct attention away from other causes. Furthermore, if a person avoids foods for a prolonged period of time, they run the risk of losing tolerance to those foods and finds that they react adversely when they try to eat them again later. So many "doctors" do not appreciate the fundamental role of food in health and disease, and tend to toss out directives about diet without being adequately qualified to do so. The fact that you have lost 30 lbs. in 6 months is very worrying.

I wish that I could direct your treatment at this stage, but unfortunately I am not in a position to do so right now. The best I can offer is to advise you to follow my histamine-restricted diet closely, making sure that you avoid all the "restricted" foods and eat all of those "allowed".

Whatever the underlying cause of your symptoms, reducing all sources of histamine in your diet should allow you some relief of your symptoms until a definitive cause can be determined. I would also suggest that you enlist the help of a registered dietitian in formulating a diet that will avoid the histamine-associated foods but provide complete balanced nutrition from alternate sources.

The dietitian should also be able to suggest an appropriate nutritional supplement if this is necessary. I am a little concerned about your daily vitamin B+C, which could have an adverse effect: B vitamins are typically derived from yeast (*Saccharomyces* species), and vitamin C might be citric acid, both of which are contraindicated on a histamine-restricted diet. You might tolerate the B vitamins, many people do, but make sure that the vitamin C is ascorbic, rather than citric acid. Your calcium and D3 supplement should be fine.

Fatigue

Question:

"Over the past 20 years, I have intermittently suffered with bouts of severe fatigue, where my glands also felt swollen around my neck and at the back, with shooting pains in my head sometimes. A few years ago, it was so severe that, after successive blood tests showing nothing I was about to be sent down the route of CFS ("Chronic Fatigue Syndrome") diagnosis—although I was constantly told it was probably depression and that I should take anti-depressants.

I have always thought it might be food related; through trial and error I've identified the following triggers: soy, miso, cinnamon, smoked salmon, Parma ham, certain cheeses, some dessert wines and Prosecco. Does this sound like it could be a response to histamine?"

Dr. Joneja replies:

There are two distinct parts to your question: the first relating to your clinical symptoms; the second to your observations regarding your response to specific foods. In neither case is it possible for me to answer definitively because I do not have details of your medical history, nor the results of any tests you may have undergone. Having said that, I will discuss both questions in light of their possible relationship to histamine intolerance.

Severe fatigue, swollen glands and shooting pains in your head as isolated symptoms do not suggest either food allergy or histamine intolerance. I am assuming that your doctors have considered other diagnoses. Sometimes blood tests alone are inadequate and more extensive investigations are required to determine possible causes. I would encourage you to seek further help in looking for the underlying mechanism for these symptoms. Too often "depression" or "psychosomatic illness" are suggested as causes for conditions that are not identifiable by standard blood tests. Continue to pursue a definitive diagnosis and do not accept this facile dismissal without further investigations if your symptoms continue to be a significant problem.

You have stated that "through trial and error" you have determined soy, miso, cinnamon, smoked salmon, Parma ham, cheeses, Prosecco and some wines to be triggers for your symptoms. These foods, as you are aware, are all likely to increase histamine, and if you are indeed histamine-sensitive, you could expect your symptoms to increase after consuming these foods. However, histamine sensitivity or intolerance is unlike allergy in that an immediate reaction to a histamine-containing or releasing food is not to be expected. The level of histamine in the body builds up over time (usually hours) and when it exceeds your individual limit of tolerance ("the level above which you develop symptoms") you will experience signs of histamine excess. Consuming a single histamine-rich food will not result in immediate symptoms, as one would expect with a typical food allergy.

To find out whether your symptoms are related to histamine intolerance, you need to follow my histamine-restricted diet closely for two to four weeks. If your symptoms remit you may assume that indeed you are histamine-sensitive and will need to follow a histamine-restricted diet for the long term. It is not possible to make a diagnosis of histamine intolerance merely on the observations that histamine-associated foods seem to trigger a reaction. I do hope that this is helpful in your quest for good health.

Hormone Fluctuations, Periods and Ovulation ("Time of the Month")

Question:

"I have been able to get my histamine level and symptoms under control with the exception of the few days around ovulation and right before my period starts. Diet and supplements aren't enough to prevent the increase in symptoms and I am wondering if there are any tips, tricks or advice that addresses the hormonal fluctuations that occur at those times of the month. I would so happy if I could avoid those monthly flare ups."

Dr. Joneja replies:

It is good to hear that you have been able to manage your symptoms by controlling your histamine level. As you are aware, hormonal fluctuations contribute quite significantly to histamine sensitivity, as estrogen and progesterone influence histamine metabolism. Both hormone levels change at ovulation and just prior to the onset of menstruation and many women experience an increase in histamine, and therefore occurrence or worsening of symptoms, at those times. Often, a histamine-restricted diet is not adequate in keeping histamine levels below a person's limit of tolerance ("the level above which symptoms appear") when endogenous histamine ("histamine produced within the body") rises significantly.

At these times you might try controlling your symptoms of histamine excess with an antihistamine. The most effective antihistamine for an acute reaction is Benadryl; however, this tends to be sedating and may not suit your lifestyle. You might find that one of the long-acting, non-sedating antihistamines such as Claritin, Sudafed or Reactine will answer your purpose.

In addition, if you are not taking a diamine oxidase (DAO) supplement as part of your histamine-controlling regimen, you might try it as an adjunct during your "reactive" periods. However, DAO acts on histamine in the digestive tract—it is not absorbed into the body, and therefore it will have very little effect in controlling endogenous histamine. Nevertheless, the enzyme might breakdown any histamine within the digestive tract, and thus add another level of histamine control. If you are taking DAO regularly, you might try increasing the dosage at times when you expect symptoms to appear.

Unfortunately, until we know a great deal more about histamine production and breakdown than we do at present, there is not a lot more that you can do to control your monthly histamine increase.

Idiopathic Anaphylaxis ("Unknown Allergy")

Question:

"I'm female, 32 years old and nearly two years ago I started waking up around 5am having anaphylaxis reactions, including stomach cramping, diarrhea, swelling of tongue, lips, tingling hands. Allergy testing has shown that I am not allergic to anything, and blood tests are also clear. I've been told it is idiopathic anaphylaxis. Could it be histamine intolerance?"

Dr. Joneja replies:

A diagnosis of idiopathic anaphylaxis means that you are experiencing symptoms typical of an anaphylactic reaction, but your doctors and other health care providers have been unable to detect any cause. You state that allergy testing has all been negative. However, as you will see from my other case studies, there are several causes for the symptoms you are experiencing including mastocytosis/mast cell activation disorders among others. I hope that all these have been considered; if not I would suggest that appropriate investigations should be undertaken as soon as possible.

If these investigations are all negative, it would be worthwhile to investigate the possibility that you are indeed experiencing histamine sensitivity as a result of a deficiency in the enzymes that break down excess histamine, especially diamine oxidase (DAO). Although "histamine excess" can have several different causes, the most important feature of them all is that an overload of histamine is responsible for the symptoms. Consequently, the histamine-restricted diet should lead to resolution, or significant reduction, in the severity of the symptoms if indeed histamine sensitivity is an issue.

In addition to the obvious causes of histamine excess, such as allergy, autoimmune diseases, chronic inflammation, mastocytosis, and DAO deficiency, several situations can increase histamine. Two of the most common are hormonal fluctuations, especially in estrogen and progesterone levels, and stress. From your description of the onset and course of your symptoms it is possible that either or both of these may be contributing. The fact that you experience symptoms at about 5.00–6.00 AM further suggests histamine build-up in excess of your limit of tolerance as it takes time for this to occur; as we have discussed, histamine levels build over hours, unlike allergic reactions where symptoms appear immediately.

I would strongly urge you to follow my histamine-restricted diet for a trial period. If your symptoms resolve or significantly improve on this regimen it would be advisable for you to follow the diet for the long term.

Interstitial Cystitis and Mast Cells

Question:

"I am a 41-year-old female, wondering if there is a possible link between histamine intolerance, interstitial cystitis (IC), and estrogen. I was diagnosed with IC 12 years ago after various bouts of UTIs and then multiple yeast infections due to the antibiotics used; I also had a sharp drop in libido.

I recently tried to take estrogen for my libido and my bladder pain and frequency increased almost immediately. I noticed I would sneeze like crazy, have itchy eyes, be angry at nothing and then the IC would act up. If I took the estrogen concurrently with Loratidine the pain was reduced. I wonder if I am having a very strong histamine response to estrogen, and whether some people with IC are really very histamine intolerant and that their estrogen is driving their pain? Also, does progesterone quell histamine release?"

Dr. Joneja Replies:

Interstitial cystitis (IC) is usually defined as a sterile (i.e. no evidence of an infective microorganism) bladder condition occurring primarily in females. Its characteristic symptoms include frequent urination, frequent wakening to urinate during the night ("nocturia"), and pain, often severe, in the pubic region. IC symptoms are often worse during ovulation and stress. The most prevalent theories to explain the pathophysiology of IC appear to be altered bladder lining and increased number of activated bladder mast cells.

The first step of the disease is thought to be the loss of the glycosaminoglycan (GAG) mucous layer, which acts as a protective barrier in the intact lining of the bladder. Reasons for the loss of this protective layer include inflammation, which might result from recurrent or chronic bladder infections among other causes. A defective bladder glycosaminoglycan (GAG) layer could allow penetration of allergens, chemicals, food preservatives, drugs, toxins, and bacteria, all of which can activate bladder mast cells.

Mast cells have been studied extensively for their involvement in allergic reactions, where they secrete numerous powerful mediators such as histamine, enzymes, leukotrienes and prostaglandins in response to immunoglobulin E (IgE) and specific allergens. However, they are also triggered by neuropeptides and have been found in close contact with neurons in the lining of the digestive tract and bladder. In conditions such as irritable bowel syndrome (IBS) and bladder conditions such as IC, mast cells appear to be activated by agents such as allergens and other triggers (listed above) which enter via a non-intact barrier lining, as well as by neurogenic factors.

When mast cells are degranulated ("release the inflammatory chemicals stored in granules") by allergic or neurogenic activation, the enzyme tryptase can be detected and is an indicator that mast cells are involved in the reaction. In IC, urine tryptase is elevated, confirming the role of mast cells in the condition. Mast cell-derived enzymes can cause tissue damage, which further exacerbates the situation by allowing the ingress of additional mast cell activating factors.

Mast cell activation is known to be enhanced by estradiol, which is a specific form of estrogen. Human bladder mast cells express estrogen receptors, which means that estrogen can attach to molecules on the mast cell surface and aid in the degranulation process and release of the stored inflammatory mediators. In contrast, bladder mast cells have very few receptors for progesterone. Research has indicated that progesterone has an inhibitory effect on the release of histamine from mast cells, even when they are stimulated by allergens or other molecules that trigger degranulation. This research tends to explain the worsening of IC symptoms during ovulation, when estrogen levels rise, and to some extent the decrease in symptoms of allergy during pregnancy when estrogen is lower and progesterone predominates.

Furthermore, acute psychological stress leads to mast cell degranulation via neurotransmitters. These findings suggest that IC could be a syndrome with neural, immune, and endocrine components, in which activated mast cells play a central role. In this respect it might be considered that interstitial cystitis should be included in the catalogue of mast cell activation disorders (MCADs).

So, with that explanation, you will be able to understand why you have experienced the reactions you report as a consequence of your frequent UTIs, estrogen supplements, as well as undoubted psychological stress. It is not possible for you to be intolerant of your own estrogen, as you seem to suspect, so that should not be a concern for you.

Of course, the next question is, "What can be done about all this to offer you some relief of your distressing symptoms?"

First, it is important for you to *avoid* increasing your estrogen levels by supplemental estrogen. The symptoms you experienced when you did try this were a result of mast cell degranulation and release of histamine, as well as other mediators.

Histamine and other mediators released from mast cells are the cause of the miserable symptoms of the condition because mast cells are central to the inflammatory process in IC. Reducing the level of histamine in your body by avoiding all sources of histamine that you can control by following a histamine-restricted diet will afford you a measure of relief. However, because other mediators in addition to histamine are involved, controlling histamine alone will not completely alleviate your symptoms. Nevertheless, I would recommend a trial on my histamine-restricted diet.

You should also try a DAO supplement; however, please understand that DAO alone will not reduce your histamine level sufficiently; it must be used as an adjunct to a histamine-restricted diet to provide optimal effects.

A small number of preliminary studies are suggesting that healing of the barrier cell layer of the bladder by replenishing the GAG in the lining of the bladder might help reduce access by foreign agents such as allergens and other mast cell activating factors. So far, the best results were obtained with 0.2% chondroitin sulphate. It might be a good idea for you to speak to your doctor about trying this approach.

Pregnancy

Question:

"The only times in my life that I felt like a normal person were the four times that I was pregnant. I was never sick or even tired; I felt wonderful. Six weeks after the birth, my old tiredness and weakness came back to stay. I've told doctors for years about this with no response. Also, at times, my ears get red and very hot. Could these things possibly have any connection to a histamine problem?"

Dr. Joneja Replies:

Most definitely: the placenta makes a significant amount of diamine oxidase (DAO) which is the most important of the enzymes that break down excess histamine in the body. DAO is made in several different organs, including the jejunum and ileum in the small intestine, kidneys, and thymus.

It is thought that the DAO made by the placenta is nature's way of protecting the developing fetus in utero. The mother benefits from this additional source of DAO while she is pregnant, and many women with histamine sensitivity as a result of DAO deficiency report feeling extremely well during their pregnancy. However, sadly their symptoms of histamine intolerance return to their pre-pregnancy intensity once the DAO from the placenta is no longer available to them.

Similarly, some women find that their allergies improve significantly while they are pregnant, as the increased level of DAO breaks down the excess histamine released in the allergic response. One of my colleagues who suffered from allergies and DAO deficiency was always delighted when she became pregnant as she could look forward to nine months of allergy relief, which she was unable to achieve at any other time.

Your red, hot ears are another sign that you are experiencing excess histamine. Histamine is a vasodilator, which means that the blood vessels widen in response to the histamine, increasing the flow of blood, often to the peripheries of the body. In your case, your ears. We see this phenomenon often in allergic children. Their red ears indicate an allergic reaction with the release of histamine affecting the area.

You will benefit from following a histamine-restricted diet. I feel sure that you will experience an increase in energy and well-being once your whole body histamine falls to a "normal" level. You may benefit from taking a DAO supplement to increase your body's ability to break down excess histamine. However, DAO supplements alone will not lower your histamine level sufficiently to allow you to become symptom-free without a corresponding reduction in your total load of histamine, which you can achieve by restricting your intake of histamine-rich and histamine-releasing foods.

Puberty, Headaches and Urticaria ("Hives")

Question:

"Recently, while on holiday in the United States, my 14-year-old daughter (who has food allergies to fish, nuts, sesame and shellfish, to name a few) had a very strange reaction. She broke out in hives all over her legs so, at the time, I gave her Benadryl. The hives came back every five hours in different locations on her legs and then arms. I took her to an allergist who said he thought it was viral and prescribed 20mg of Reactine daily. She has been on Reactine for 10 days; she is extremely fatigued and has had a constant (and at times, severe) headache. When I lower the dose of Reactine, in hopes it might alleviate her headache, her face begins flushing.

Although she has allergies, she has never experienced hives or headaches in the past. Just as a note she has just started to menstruate. Could you give me some insight into whether you think this reaction could be an allergy, viral or histamine related?"

Dr. Joneja Replies:

It is not uncommon for a girl entering menarche ("onset of puberty") to experience symptoms of histamine excess such as hives, flushing, headaches and fatigue. Although the precise mechanism of the association is still unclear, research is indicating that histamine levels are influenced by hormones, especially progesterone and estrogen, which change significantly during the menstrual cycle. For some reason, the changes in the level of these hormones at menarche and menopause seem to result in unusually high levels of histamine release. These effects seem to be diminished over time as the body adjusts to the changes.

Because your daughter is atopic—in other words, is already sensitized to several allergens—she is at a higher than normal risk for developing symptoms of histamine excess because her basal level of histamine is already unusually high. Even a slight change, probably triggered by hormone production during her menstrual cycle, will cause her "histamine bucket" to overflow.

Of course there is the possibility that your daughter contracted a viral infection during her holiday in the USA, which would increase her histamine levels as any infection would, because it is an inflammatory reaction which inevitably results in histamine release. If this is the case, her symptoms will diminish as the virus is cleared from her body.

In any event, whether your daughter's symptoms are due to an infection, allergy, or hormonal fluctuations, she is dealing with an excess of histamine. The effects can be controlled by antihistamines such as Benadryl, which however, is a sedative and therefore will increase her fatigue, or a non-sedating antihistamine such as Reactine.

For the long-term I would suggest that she follow my histamine-restricted diet, making sure that she consumes all of the "allowed foods" to ensure complete balanced nutrition, which is critical at this stage of her development. The diet will at least reduce the exogenous ("from outside the body") sources, so decreasing the total body level of histamine. In addition, supplementary diamine oxidase, taken immediately before food, will aid in breaking down any histamine in a meal before it enters the body.

It is most likely that as your daughter's body adjusts to the hormonal changes, her histamine levels will return to a more "normal" level and her present symptoms will resolve to a large extent. I hope that it will be of some reassurance to you both to know that the situation is temporary and should not be a long-term issue. However, the adjustment period is an individual characteristic, so unfortunately I cannot give you any time frame in which to expect such an improvement.

Sexual issues: semen allergy and vaginal irritation

Question:

"I have had an extreme bout of vaginal irritation since I started consuming kefir. I have since stopped but it continues to plague me. I also used to get headaches when I drank kombucha or ate pickles, olives etc.

I'm also concerned about allergies to semen. My problems seem to worsen when I have been intimate with my partner of 9 years. It had never been a problem before. Would that be due to a high histamine diet on his part and my reacting to that or have you found any other connection?"

Dr. Joneja Replies:

This is a very intriguing question encompassing several different points, which will allow me to discuss a number of facts and misconceptions about histamine intolerance. However, you do not provide your age, I have no information on your recent medical history, and you do not state how long the symptoms you report have been a problem. So I shall use your questions to discuss each aspect of the subject in general terms.

First of all, vaginal irritation *on its own* does not suggest histamine intolerance or sensitivity. It is more likely to be a result of a vaginal yeast infection (candidiasis or moniliasis). Do you have a vaginal discharge, and have you consulted your doctor about this? If this is not the case, a reaction to your partner's semen, as you have suspected, may be the cause (see below).

Acidophilus is the species name of *Lactobacillus acidophilus*, a bacterium often used in making yogurt, and kefir among other products. It is the fermenting agent in acidophilus milk. Although it does contribute to the histamine level in fermented products, consuming kefir alone will be insufficient to raise your histamine level into the symptomatic range (that is, exceeding your limit of tolerance) unless you are consuming several sources of histamine at the same time, or are experiencing a reaction that increases the release of histamine in your body. This could be allergy, or a number of other conditions that involve inflammation.

Your experience of headaches after consuming kombucha, pickles, olives etc. does point to excess histamine as a cause, since these contain fairly high levels of histamine. It would be worthwhile for you to follow a histamine-restricted diet in order to determine whether histamine sensitivity is indeed causing or contributing to your symptoms. Provided allergy is not an issue you might also find DAO supplements helpful.

The question as to whether you can react to your partner consuming a high histamine diet indicates a misconception about histamine intolerance. Histamine sensitivity, or intolerance is not an allergy. You cannot react by contact. If someone consumes a high histamine diet, the histamine is present in their blood plasma; it cannot be transmitted to, nor affect anyone else. Your partner would develop symptoms if he has histamine intolerance, but even then, his reactions would not affect you.

In searching the internet, you might find some rather fascinating theories suggesting that the high stress involved in sexual intercourse might release histamine, and account for the flushing that some women experience. However, there is no evidence-based research data to suggest that such "positive stress" can influence histamine levels in either partner.

The only reliable research has been carried out in men. In a study[1] to evaluate the course of histamine plasma levels through different stages of sexual arousal in healthy male subjects, histamine slightly decreased in the local blood when the penis became tumescent. During rigidity, histamine decreased further but remained unaltered in the phase of detumescence and after ejaculation. In the systemic circulation, no alterations were observed with the initiation or termination of penile erection, whereas a significant drop was registered following ejaculation.

The researchers concluded that the results were not in favor of the hypothesis of an excitatory role of histamine in the control of penile erection. Unfortunately, at present we do not have any reliable research on histamine levels in women during intercourse.

As you have suggested, your vaginal irritation could be the result of an allergy to your partner's semen. If semen allergy is present, the woman should not have any symptoms when she and her partner use a condom. The allergic reaction should only happen during unprotected sex. To confirm the allergy, an allergist or gynecologist can carry out skin tests using your partner's semen as the allergen.

It would be worthwhile for you to consult a suitably qualified practitioner for a definitive diagnosis. In advising women with semen allergy in my practice (of which there have been very few; in my experience it is a rare condition), I have found that douching with alkaline salts prior to intercourse has worked amazingly well, especially in cases where the couple is trying to become pregnant or do not wish to use condoms.

Recipe for alkaline salts:

Mix sodium bicarbonate and potassium bicarbonate in a 2:1 ratio:
1 cup sodium bicarbonate/baking soda
½ cup potassium bicarbonate (available from a compounding pharmacy or on the internet)

Add 1 tablespoon of the mixture to ½ cup warm water.
Use as required prior to intercourse.

Urticaria ("Hives"), Stress and Depression

Question:

"I am 18 years old and have had chronic hives over my whole body since I was about 1-year-old. The attacks have increased over time and are mainly at night.

Allergy prick tests haven't shown anything major, except slight evidence of seasonal allergies and dog dander. An immunology specialist that it could be an autoimmune condition and to treat it symptomatically. I have been taking Zyrtec daily, often laced with Benadryl.

I also have moderate OCD with bouts of depression and anxiety. In the past year I have also acquired a low grade vaginal yeast infection that is not clearing with treatment.

Can you please explain why do I break out mainly in the middle of the night-to-morning? Also, my therapist has suggested that I take an anti-anxiety pill to take the 'edge' off. Could OCD, depression and anxiety fuel the histamine problem, or does histamine contribute to roller coaster anxiety and depression?

I have an appointment with a new allergist soon; can you please suggest the tests that I might expect him to perform?"

Dr. Joneja Replies:

You have provided some interesting pieces of information that may offer some answers as to the origin of your chronic urticaria ("hives"), your depression and anxiety, and even perhaps the reason why your yeast infection seems resistant to treatment.

As you will be aware, histamine plays a key role in urticaria. Histamine causes an increased permeability of small blood vessels, which allows fluid to move from the cells into tissues. This causes the slight swelling and reddening typical of the urticarial lesions. Hives are always itchy, which is one of the indicators that excess histamine is present. An important question here is: what is the origin of your excess histamine? Hives are frequently part of an allergic reaction as histamine is released whenever mast cells discharge their inflammatory mediators in the allergic response. However, you indicate that allergy tests in the past were rather uninformative, so an allergic reaction may not be the main cause of your hives.

The immunologist you consulted may be correct in suggesting an autoimmune reaction, but until now it would appear that this has not been confirmed, neither has any specific autoimmune disease been diagnosed.

Obsessive-compulsive disorder (OCD) and anxiety are highly stressful reactions. There are very close associations between stress and the immune system; these interactions are becoming more completely understood as research into the physiological processes is evolving. A high level of stress initiates activation of two nervous system responses:

- The hypothalamic-pituitary adrenal axis response that is responsible for the "fight or flight' reaction of the central nervous system involving the release of cortisol
- The sympathetic nervous system that results in release of neurotransmitters such as epinephrine ("adrenalin"), noradrenalin and dopamine ("catecholamines").

In both cases, mediators generated in these reactions initiate responses in the immune system, involving T-cells, cytokines and mast cells.

However, each of the processes can have different effects on the immune system: cortisol tends to *suppress* the immune response, leading to an increased risk of infections as well as other physiological imbalances and additional triggers from the sympathetic nervous system can *activate* the immune response and lead to degranulation of mast cells and release of inflammatory mediators, including histamine. Furthermore, the two processes can influence each other, setting up a kind of cyclical effect. Unfortunately, at present there is still much for us to learn about how these processes result in reactions and symptoms in individuals. It is often not possible to predict exactly how the immune system will respond to the different kinds of stress that as humans we are constantly experiencing.

So—a rather long and complex answer to your question, but I do hope that an understanding of the processes that may be going on your body will help you to feel more in control.

It is certainly possible that excess histamine is playing an important role in your symptoms, both as a trigger for your chronic hives, and as a possible mediator of your OCD, anxiety and other nervous system reactions, as well as a possible consequence of them. Understanding is the first stage—the next question, of course, is what can you do about it?

You indicate that you will be consulting an allergist shortly. It would be informative if he or she orders blood tests for IgE-mediated allergy, and if positive, management strategies can be initiated to deal with them. In addition, if the allergist is a clinical immunologist perhaps investigation of a possible underlying autoimmune process may be useful. Unfortunately, in my experience, chronic hives is frequently labelled "idiopathic urticaria" (in other words, "cause unknown") and no further investigations are carried out.

As for the OCD and anxiety: there is not a lot that can be done at this stage in our knowledge to address the possible reactions that are taking place; however, I suggest that a trial on a histamine-restricted diet will definitely demonstrate whether excess histamine is involved in your adverse reactions and controlling that may provide some relief of all of your symptoms.

You ask why your symptoms occur most noticeably from the middle of the night to morning. Two reasons: histamine from your diet will build up during the day and may "overflow your histamine bucket". Furthermore, there is a type of circadian rhythm associated with histamine release and breakdown within the body; we need histamine for several essential functions, so it will be constantly synthesized ("manufactured or produced") by body cells over the course of a 24-hour period.

Experiments with rats indicate that histamine release gradually increases in the second half of the light period (2.00–8.00 PM) and the average histamine release during the dark period (8.00 PM–8.00 AM) is significantly higher than that during the light period. This clear change in histamine release suggests that the histamine-producing process is related to the circadian rhythm . Although it is not yet known exactly how this works in humans, in your case histamine is reaching its optimal production during the night, and so overwhelms the enzymes that break it down (mainly diamine oxidase DAO) and symptoms of histamine excess develop.

ABOUT DR. JANICE VICKERSTAFF JONEJA, PH.D.

Dr. Janice Joneja is a researcher, educator, author, and clinical counsellor with over 30 years of experience in the area of biochemical and immunological reactions involved in food allergy and intolerances. Dr. Joneja holds a Ph.D. in medical microbiology and immunology and was a registered dietitian (RD) for 27 years.

She has been a member of the faculty at several Canadian universities, starting her career as an Assistant Professor in the Department of Microbiology, Faculty of Science, and in the Faculty of Dentistry, at the University of British Columbia, Vancouver. Since 2001, Dr. Joneja has been a faculty member in the School of Biomedical and Molecular Sciences, at the University of Surrey, in England, teaching in the M.Sc. course in Nutritional Medicine. For 12 years, she was head of the Allergy Nutrition Program at the Vancouver Hospital and Health Sciences Centre.

Dr. Joneja is the author of eight books and dietetic practice manuals on food allergy, a textbook on Irritable Bowel Syndrome, and several distance education courses. Her most recent books include "The Health Professional's Guide to Food Allergies and Intolerances", "Dealing with Food Allergies", and "Dealing with Food Allergies in Babies and Children". You can find Dr. Joneja's books on Amazon.

Dr. Joneja's work has been published in peer-reviewed scientific and medical journals, as well as in popular magazines. She is a respected lecturer at universities, colleges and hospitals internationally, and regularly appears on television and radio call-in shows as an expert in her field.

Dr. Joneja is President of Vickerstaff Health Services, Inc., a practice that provides counselling for people suffering from all aspects of adverse reactions to food, and resources for the professionals and care-givers who support them.

FURTHER RESOURCES

You can find more of Dr. Joneja's books on Amazon:
www.amazon.com / www.amazon.co.uk / www.amazon.ca

A companion volume: "Histamine Intolerance: the Complete Guide for Medical Professionals" will be published in Autumn 2017.

At the time of writing, there is only one food-grade DAO supplement available: Umbrellux DAO (www.umbrellux.com)

The case studies in this book were first published on Foods Matter (www.foodsmatter.com); a website dedicated to freefrom living, food allergy and intolerance, and Celiac disease.

REFERENCES

What is Histamine and Histamine Intolerance?

General references for this section

Joneja Vickerstaff JM. Dealing with Food Allergies: A Practical Guide to Detecting Culprit Foods and Eating a Healthy, Enjoyable Diet. Boulder: Bull Publishing Company; 2003. p. 233–246.

Joneja Vickerstaff JM. The Health Professional's Guide to Food Allergies and Intolerances. Chicago: Academy of Nutrition and Dietetics; 2012. Chapter 31: Histamine Sensitivity; p. 291–304.

Joneja JMV, Carmona Silva C. Outcome of a histamine-restricted diet based on chart audit. J Nutr Environ Med. 2001;11(4):249–262.

Specific references for this section

[1] Maintz L, Novak N. Histamine and histamine intolerance. Am J Clin Nutr. 2007;85:1185–1196.

[2] Huertz GN, Schwelberger HG. Simultaneous purification of the histamine degrading enzymes diamine oxidase and histamine N-methyltransferase from the same tissue. Inflamm Res. 2003;52(suppl 1):S65-S66.

[3] Wohrl S, Hemmer W, Focke M, Rappersberger K, Jarische R. Histamine intolerance-like symptoms in healthy volunteers after oral provocation with liquid histamine. Allergy Asthma Proc. 2004;25:305-311.

[4] Castells MC. Mastocytosis: classification, diagnosis, and clinical presentation. Allergy Asthma Proc. 2004;25:33–36.

[5] Friere M, Patel R, Celestin J. Mast cell activation syndrome: a review.

Curr Allergy Asthma Rep. 2013 Feb;13(1):27-32.

[6] Maintz L, Schwartzer V, Bieber T, van der Ven K, Novak N. Effects of histamine and diamine oxidase activities on pregnancy: a critical review. Hum Reprod Update. 2008;14(5):485-495.

[7] Swiss Interest Group Histamine Intolerance (SIGHI). *Medicaments.* Available from: http://www.histaminintoleranz.ch/en/therapy_medicaments.html [Accessed 31st January 2017].

[8] Dyer J, Warren K, Merlin S, Metcalfe DD, Kaliner M. Measurement of plasma histamine: description of an improved method and normal values. J Allergy Clin Imunol. 1982;70:72-87.

Managing Histamine Intolerance

General references for this section

Joneja Vickerstaff JM. Dealing with Food Allergies: A Practical Guide to Detecting Culprit Foods and Eating a Healthy, Enjoyable Diet. Boulder: Bull Publishing Company; 2003. p. 233–246.

Joneja Vickerstaff JM. Food Allergies and Intolerances: Client Education Tools for Dietary Management. Chicago: Academy of Nutrition and Dietetics; 2013.

Joneja Vickerstaff JM. The Health Professional's Guide to Food Allergies and Intolerances. Chicago: Academy of Nutrition and Dietetics; 2012.

References for Case Studies

Anaphylaxis

[1] Hershko AY, Dranitzki Z, Ulmanski R, Levi-Schaffer F, Naparstek Y. Constitutive hyperhistaminaemia: a possible mechanism for recurrent anaphylaxis. Scand J Clin Lab Invest. 2001;61:449–452.

General reference for Anxiety

Joneja JMV, Carmona Silva C. Outcome of a histamine-restricted diet based on chart audit. J Nutr Environ Med. 2001;11(4):249–262.

Interstitial Cystitis and Mast Cells

Muñoz-Cruz S, Mendoza-Rodríguez Y, Nava-Castro KE, Yepez-Mulia L, Morales-Montor J. Gender-related effects of sex steroids on histamine release and FcεRI expression in rat peritoneal mast cells. J Immunol Res [journal on the Internet]. 2015;2015(1):Article 351829. Available from: http://www.ncbi.nlm.nih.gov/pmc/articles/PMC4417946/pdf/JIR2015-351829.pdf

Whitmore K, Theoharides TC. When to suspect interstitial cystitis. J Fam Pract. 2011 Jun;60(6):340–348.

Theoharides TC, Pang X, Letourneau R, Sant GR. Interstitial cystitis: a neuroimmunoendocrine disorder. Ann N Y Acad Sci. 1998 May;840:619–634.

Theoharides TC, Alysandratos KD, Angelidou A, Delivanis DA, Sismanopoulos N, Zhang B, et al. Mast cells and inflammation. Biochim Biophys Acta. 2012 Jan;1822(1):21–33.

Vasiadi M, Kempuraj D, Boucher W, Kalogeromitros D, Theoharides TC. Progesterone inhibits mast cell secretion. Int J Immunopathol Pharmacol. 2006 Oct–Dec;19(4):787–794.

Vliagoftis H, Dimitriadou V, Boucher W, Rozniecki JJ, Correia I, Raam S, et al. Estradiol augments while tamoxifen inhibits rat mast cell secretion. Int Arch Allergy Immunol. 1992;98(4):398–409.

Sexual Issues

[1]Uckert S, Wilken M, Stief C, Trottmann M, Kuczyk M, Becker A. Is there a significance of histamine in the control of the human male sexual response? *Andrologia* 2012 May;44 Suppl 1:538–542.

Urticaria, Stress and Depression

Mochizuki T, Yamatodani A, Okakuta K, Horii A, Inagaki N, Wada H. Circadian rhythm of histamine release from the hypothalamus of freely moving rats. Physiol Behav. 1992 Feb;51(2): 391–394.

INDEX

allergic reaction, 2, 4, 5, 8, 9, 15, 40, 43, 48, 53, 57, 65, 66, 70, 75, 77

allergy / allergen, v, 3, 4, 8, 10, 13, 15, 16, 18, 38, 43, 50, 53, 56, 58, 61, 64, 66, 70, 73, 76

allergy, food, v, 8, 15, 40, 48, 61, 83

anaphylaxis, 47, 53, 57, 64

antihistamines, 16, 18, 44, 49, 52, 56, 63, 71, 76

anxiety, 2, 38, 45, 52, 57, 76

artificial colors, 7, 11, 24, 27, 29, 35

asthma, 47

autoimmune conditions, 13, 38, 65, 76, 77, 79

autoimmune disease, 8

autoimmune reaction, 77

bacteria, 1, 10, 23, 50, 66

blood pressure, drop in / hypotension, 2, 47, 54

breathing difficulties, 2, 38, 43, 51

bucket (of histamine), 3, 4, 7, 9, 15, 16, 18, 23, 39, 51, 71, 79

celiac disease, 47, 83

chest pain, 2, 38

children, 22, 70

Chronic Fatigue Syndrome, 60

conjunctivitis, 2

consciousness, loss of, 2

DAO / Diamine Oxidase, 3, 4, 6, 7, 13, 14, 16, 17, 19, 20, 22, 36, 48, 51, 55, 57, 63, 64, 68, 69, 72, 74, 79, 83

degranulation, 43, 67, 78

depression, 45, 60, 61, 76

diabetes, 44, 47, 49

diarrhea, 45, 64

digestion, 8, 51

digestive problems (heartburn, indigestion, reflux), 2, 19, 47

digestive tract, 1, 4, 16, 20, 43, 45, 50, 63, 66

disturbed sensation, 45

dizziness, 38

EpiPen, 52

estrogen, 14, 51, 55, 59, 63, 65, 71

fatigue, 38, 60, 71, 72

FGIDs / functional gastrointestinal disorders, 45, 46

flushing / reddening of the skin, 1, 4, 49, 71, 74

food intolerance, 40, 83

food preservatives, 7, 11, 24, 27, 29, 33, 35, 36, 66

food, histamine-releasing, 12, 37

food, histamine-rich, 7, 9, 10, 15, 17, 22, 45

headaches / migraines, 2, 4, 38, 70, 73

heart, racing / tachycardia, 2, 47, 54

histamine-restricted diet, 7, 8, 13, 14, 16, 17, 18, 22, 24, 36, 39, 44, 46, 48, 52, 55, 56, 59, 62, 63, 64, 68, 70, 72, 74, 79

hives / urticaria, 1, 47, 49, 53, 54, 71, 76, 79

HNMT / histamine N-methyltransferase, 3, 51, 57

hormones, 4, 6, 14, 51, 55, 59, 62, 65, 71, 72

IBS, 45, 67

immune system, 1, 4, 5, 8, 40, 51, 54, 77

inflammation, 4, 5, 6, 13, 19, 38, 44, 45, 48, 54, 56, 59, 65, 66, 72, 74, 77

interstitial cystitis, 65, 67

itching / pruritus, 1, 46, 49, 52, 65, 77

limit of tolerance (histamine), 3, 15, 16, 17, 23, 37, 39, 41, 52, 62, 63, 65, 74

mast cells / leukocytes, 5, 18,